AXA Equitable Life Insurance Company (NY, NY) - Retirement

The Members Retirement Program, administered by AXA [illegible] is a valuable benefit for retirement planning. [illegible] sponsored by AAMA exclusively for its members since 1970. Built from the ground up to meet the specific needs of members, the retirement program PROVIDES THE OPPORTUNITY to build your retirement assets with ease and affordability.

AXA Equitable is proud to be an EXPERIENCED PROVIDER of retirement planning solutions for small businesses, especially ones [illegible] and has presented as [illegible] members with innovative retirement strategies for more than 45 years. Our retirement solutions are DESIGNED to meet the needs of business owners at every stage of the way.

At AXA Equitable, our GOAL is to help deliver retirement solutions defined by your [illegible] to accomplish [illegible] complimentary [illegible] comparison of your existing plan, contact a knowledgeable Retirement Program Specialist at 800-523-1125 [illegible] or VISIT US at www.axa-[illegible]plan.com.

GE-[illegible]

The Members Retirement Program [illegible] is funded by a group [illegible] issued and distributed by AXA Equitable Life Insurance Company, NY, NY [illegible] restrictions, fees and [illegible] please see the [illegible] information [illegible].

Be a Champion

80 TIPS

to Work Smarter, Save Money, and Show the Love to Clients and Pets

American Animal Hospital Association Press
12575 West Bayaud Avenue
Lakewood, Colorado 80228
800-252-2242 or 303-986-2800
press.aaha.org

AAHA press

ISBN 13: 978-1-53826-253-5

Library of Congress Cataloging-in-Publication Data is available at the Library of Congress.

Developmental Editor: Bess Maher
Managing Editor: Laura Esterman
Associate Production Editor: Karie Simpson
Interior Designer: Kate Moore
Cover Designer: Kate Moore

Contents

Preface

AAHA's goal is to help all practices enhance patient care, improve client service, and create empowered and motivated teams. Our accreditation team visits more than 1,200 stellar practice teams every year. We see how top practices run things, and we are always amazed at the ingenious solutions practice teams use to make their jobs easier and patient outcomes better.

When we spot a way of doing things that is unique, clever, fun, or just plain cute, something that will improve patient care, client service, or team satisfaction, we like to share it. In this book, we've gathered the best of those tips to share with you.

Other publications go into depth about medical and management skills. That is not what we aimed to do in this book. Instead, we've compiled the little things you can do to make a big difference . . . for your staff, clients, and—most important—your patients!

Veterinary professionals are amazingly creative and dedicated to excellence. Do you have a tip or two that would help other practices shine? Share it by sending an email to practice.accreditation@aaha.org.

Debbie Gadomski
AAHA National Field Operations Manager

Acknowledgments

When our AAHA Practice Consultants are out in the field, part of their mission is to impart information—information about the AAHA Standards, medical and technical tips, and management advice. But information sharing goes both ways, and our consultants also learn from the veterinary practices they visit. And whenever they come across a particularly helpful or unique tip, they share it with our central office, which is how the idea for this book originated. Thanks go to our Practice Consultants for being attentive to the many great things our member practices do and for sharing those tips with headquarters so we could in turn share them with you.

Special thanks go to AAHA Practice Accreditation Coordinator Morgan Schneider, who worked closely with the editors at AAHA Press to fact-check and edit the tips, fleshing them out so that they would be as useful as possible to veterinary professionals.

Finally, this book would not have been possible without the smart, caring, and hardworking veterinary teams who contributed their tips to improve patient care and practice operations. The American Animal Hospital Association is honored to serve you as you serve your patients. In that spirit, we thank the following practices:

- 43rd Avenue Animal Hospital, Glendale, Arizona, accredited since 2009
- Advanced Veterinary Care, Farmington, Connecticut, accredited since 2015
- Anacapa Animal Hospital, Ventura, California, accredited since 1986
- Animal Emergency Hospital of Mansfield, Mansfield, Texas, accredited since 2012
- Animal Emergency Medical Center-Referral, Torrance, California, accredited since 2008
- Animal Family Veterinary Care Center, Davenport, Iowa, accredited since 2002
- Animal Medical Center of Chandler, Chandler, Arizona, accredited since 2014
- Animal Medical Center of Estes Park PC, Estes Park, Colorado, accredited since 1994
- Animal Medical Clinic of Gulf Gate, Sarasota, Florida, accredited since 1977
- Bear Valley Veterinary Care Center, Denver, Colorado, accredited since 1978
- Bethany Animal Hospital, Sycamore, Illinois, accredited since 1980
- Blandford Animal Hospital, Blandford, Massachusetts, accredited since 1991
- Bolton Veterinary Hospital PC, Bolton, Connecticut, accredited since 1976
- Carmel Veterinary Clinic, Carmel, Indiana, accredited since 1988
- Celtic Creatures Veterinary Clinic Ltd., Sydney, Nova Scotia, Canada, accredited since 2010
- Columbia Animal Clinic PC, Brooklyn, Michigan, accredited since 2014
- Country Doctor Veterinary Hospital, New Tripoli, Pennsylvania, accredited since 2014
- Country Hills Pet Hospital, Eden, Wisconsin, accredited since 2000

- Creature Comforts Animal Hospital, Las Vegas, Nevada, accredited since 2010
- Doctors Pet Clinic, Murrieta, California, accredited since 2014
- Dog and Cat Dentist Inc., Culver City, California, accredited since 2014
- Evans Animal Hospital, Evans, Georgia, accredited since 1988
- Gardner Animal Care Center, Gardner, Massachusetts, accredited since 2001
- Greenland Veterinary Hospital, Greenland, New Hampshire, accredited since 2014
- Guide Dogs for the Blind Inc., Boring, Oregon, accredited since 1998
- Harlingen Veterinary Clinic, Belle Mead, New Jersey, accredited since 1990
- Harmony Veterinary Center, Arvada, Colorado, accredited since 2010
- Hill Country Animal Hospital, Helotes, Texas, accredited since 2000
- Hope Springs Veterinary at Great Bridge, Chesapeake, Virginia, accredited since 1993
- Hulen Hills Animal Hospital, Fort Worth, Texas, accredited since 1984
- Jordan Creek Animal Hospital, West Des Moines, Iowa, accredited since 1994
- Knollwood Animal Hospital PC, Lake Bluff, Illinois, accredited since 1990
- Larchmont Animal Clinic, Los Angeles, California, accredited since 1981
- Markham Animal Clinic Ltd., Markham, Illinois, accredited since 1971
- Michigan City Animal Hospital, Michigan City, Indiana, accredited since 1991
- Mid-Island Animal Hospital, Hicksville, New York, accredited since 1985
- Montrose Animal Hospital, Marietta, Georgia, accredited since 2012
- Mueller Pet Medical Center, Sacramento, California, accredited since 2012
- Multnomah County Animal Services, Troutdale, Oregon, accredited since 2006
- NorthStar VETS, Robbinsville, New Jersey, accredited since 2010
- Oasis Animal Hospital, Henderson, Nevada, accredited since 2007
- Orchard Road Animal Hospital, Montgomery, Illinois, accredited since 2010
- Palo Verde Animal Hospital, Phoenix, Arizona, accredited since 1978
- Parkside Animal Care Center, Green Bay, Wisconsin, accredited since 2013
- Petaluma Veterinary Hospital, Petaluma, California, accredited since 1986
- Pets and Vets as Partners, West Lafayette, Indiana, accredited since 2012
- Pets in Need, Redwood City, California, accredited since 2014
- Pierrefonds Animal Hospital, Pierrefonds (Montreal), Quebec, accredited since 1995
- Shady Brook Animal Hospital, Magnolia, Texas, accredited since 2006
- South Carolina Veterinary Emergency Care, Columbia, South Carolina, accredited since 2003
- Stack Veterinary Hospital, Syracuse, New York, accredited since 1957
- Stone House Animal Hospital, Topeka, Kansas, accredited since 2014
- Sunnyvale Veterinary Clinic, Sunnyvale, California, accredited since 2011
- Tara Animal Hospital Inc., Colleyville, Texas, accredited since 2010
- VCA Angel Animal Hospital, Flower Mound, Texas, accredited since 2013
- VCA Animal Health Center, Clifton Park, New York, accredited since 1990
- VCA Pacific Petcare Veterinary Hospital of Carmel Valley, San Diego, California, accredited since 1995
- VCA Snohomish Animal Hospital, Snohomish, Washington, accredited since 1993
- VCA South Shore Animal Hospital #154, South Weymouth, Massachusetts, accredited since 2013
- VCA Village Animal Hospital, Palm Bay, Florida, accredited since 2010
- Veterinary Associates of Cape Cod Corp., South Yarmouth, Massachusetts, accredited since 1979
- Veterinary Medical Center of Long Island, West Islip, New York, accredited since 2012
- Walnut Grove Animal Hospital, Loganville, Georgia, accredited since 2013
- Wignall Animal Hospital, Dracut, Massachusetts, accredited since 2012
- Willowdale Animal Hospital, Willowdale, Ontario, Canada, accredited since 1974
- Windmill Animal Hospital, Abilene, Texas, accredited since 2012

Chapter 1

Organization and Efficiency

We place our **rigid** and **FLEXIBLE** endoscopy lines into corrugated CLEAR oxygen delivery tubes prior to **gas sterilization.** **This prevents the sterilization pouches from** shrinking **and** CRIMPING **the lines.** We also found it helps to keep them **NEAT** and **organized** in storage.

Animal Emergency Medical Center-Referral

Torrance, California

When sharp instruments VIBRATE against the side and bottom of the cleaning tub, it can bore TINY FISSURES IN THE TUB and degrade it. So we place the small, sharp dental instruments like dental burs and root canal files into a **stainless steel tea strainer**. This also helps us keep track of them, and allows them to be sterilized properly. We place the larger sharp dental instruments like root tip elevators and dental explorers in **glass beakers** to SHIELD the cleaning tub from direct contact.

Dog and Cat Dentist Inc.
Culver City, California

We used to spend **SO MUCH TIME** waiting for our micro slides to dry, but then we started using a **nail polish dryer**. It's much faster and easier than using a blow dryer or air drying them.

Pets and Vets as Partners
West Lafayette, Indiana

Instead of tossing out or recycling our plastic vaccine trays, we use them in our urine collection kits for pet owners. They work great since they are flat, don't absorb the urine, and have a large surface area. As an added bonus, they make it easier for clients to collect the urine, making them more compliant.

43rd Avenue Animal Hospital
Glendale, Arizona

We recently switched from keeping our vaccines in the fridge to keeping them in a vaccine chiller. We found this method of storage to be so efficient that we bought a second one for our feline vaccines. Moreover, it freed up space in the fridge.

Jordan Creek Animal Hospital
West Des Moines, Iowa

We use a **"grass"-style drying rack,** normally used for drying baby bottles, to dry our **endotracheal tubes.**

IT WORKS GREAT.

You place the tubes on the **grass** and the WATER DRAINS FROM THE TUBES to the lower tray, allowing the tubes to AIR DRY FULLY before the next use. **Plus,** the grass and tray can be cleaned in the dishwasher.

Wignall Animal Hospital
Dracut, Massachusetts

We have placed buckets filled with small pinwheels outside our practice with signs that ask, "Please place a pinwheel where your pet did its deed so our staff knows where to clean." Someone from our staff goes out every few hours and can easily spot which areas need to be tended to.

Advanced Veterinary Care
Farmington, Connecticut

Once, one of our hospitalized dogs bit through its leash on a walk and got loose. Now when we walk hospitalized dogs outside, we double leash them and carry walkie-talkies with us. The walkies allow the person outside to call for help and still be free to catch the loose dog. It gives us an added bit of security.

Anacapa Animal Hospital
Ventura, California

Being a VERY high volume shelter, adoption center, and veterinary hospital, we have a STRINGENT CLEANING PROTOCOL for our KENNELS. After we hose down, disinfect, and squeegee a run to remove any excess WATER, we use an electric leaf blower to QUICKLY and FULLY dry the runs. This extra step helps to REDUCE the humidity as well as minimize ODORS, MOLD, and BACTERIA.

Pets in Need
Redwood City, California

We were TIRED of dealing with peeling tape and a dirty-looking "white" board in our treatment area, so, like a lot of hospitals operated by VCA, we overlaid the whole board with a LARGE piece of glass. This way our whiteboard stays clean AND we don't have to deal with peeling tape.

VCA Pacific Petcare Veterinary Hospital of Carmel Valley
San Diego, California

We use thick clear shelf liner to protect our linens from contamination. We attach it to the door fronts of the upper cages where the linens are stored by using a hole punch and zip ties. None of the liner has torn yet, and it's easy to wipe down and disinfect.

Blandford Animal Hospital
Blandford, Massachusetts

We had custom pull-out shelves built around the hospital to house the doctors' laptops. The laptops fit perfectly inside them and power cords are permanently attached to each shelf. This way, the computers are always charged, easily accessible, safe, and inconspicuous.

Bolton Veterinary Hospital PC
Bolton, Connecticut

Our practice **purchased a bar code scanner** to use for all the products that we DISPENSE **or** SELL. It took a little while to get the equipment and process set up, **BUT** IT WAS WORTH THE TIME AND EFFORT. Now we always ring up the correct item, and our inventory has **little to no discrepancy.**

Animal Medical Center of Estes Park PC

Estes Park, Colorado

To help our dogs that are older, arthritic, or scared of slippery floors, we USE YOGA MATS that we were able to get as DONATIONS from a local yoga studio. To encourage the dogs to go where we want them to go, we line the mats on the floor like RUNNERS; and to keep the dogs in place, we pick up all the other mats around them so they don't have a SECURE place to move. The mats are also easy to DISINFECT.

Oasis Animal Hospital
Henderson, Nevada

We designed small caution tags such as "NO FOOD" and "SAVE URINE" to hang on kennels to help notify our staff of any patient alerts.

Jordan Creek Animal Hospital
West Des Moines, Iowa

To better transport dirty laundry through the hospital, we use a laundry basket lined with a plastic bag, and then use a large chip clip to close the bag. The plastic clips are an inexpensive way to keep the bag closed, are easy to open, and can be sterilized with a disinfectant spray.

Oasis Animal Hospital
Henderson, Nevada

We use divided lunch trays to organize catheter placement supplies for each patient and miscellaneous supplies for new puppy appointments. This method helps us visualize everything we need as well as be prepared, efficient, and organized.

Bear Valley Veterinary Care Center
Denver, Colorado

We installed a flat-screen monitor in the treatment area to display whiteboard software. In the software, we list all the patients in the hospital with color-coded dots next to their names to indicate which doctor is in charge of the case, which is then displayed on the monitor. The screen also displays pending procedures and ready-to-go status. This system helps everyone know the pertinent information about each patient, and, if there are questions, which veterinarian to ask for clarification.

VCA Angel Animal Hospital
Flower Mound, Texas

Recently, we started using two-way radios in our practice. Everyone has an assigned radio with an ear bud during office hours. Now, instead of wasting time trying to find someone, we call each other on the radio. The coverage area for the radios is about a mile, so we can even call someone out walking a dog. The radios took some time to get used to, but they made up for that in increased efficiency.

Walnut Grove Animal Hospital
Loganville, Georgia

Chapter 2

Anesthesia, Surgery, and Medication

To help avoid surgical errors, we have a special "MASS REMOVAL" intake sheet that includes marking the location of any masses on a drawing of a dog or cat, as well as OPTIONS to discard the masses, hold them for six months in formalin, or send them out for histopath. The sheet is FILLED OUT AND SIGNED BY THE OWNER AT DROP-OFF, making clear what will happen during surgery to both staff and owners.

Pierrefonds Animal Hospital
Pierrefonds (Montreal), Quebec

To raise the bar on our anesthesia and sedation TECHNIQUES, we INVITED a local board-certified veterinary anesthesiologist to come and offer suggestions for improvement. It was GREAT to hear some tips for refining our techniques, along with what we were doing well.

Guide Dogs for the Blind Inc.
Boring, Oregon

In our hospital, we use a **color-coding SYSTEM** for IV catheter placement with our surgical patients.

After we place the IV catheter, we wrap the catheter with **RED vet wrap.**

When we remove the IV catheter, we wrap the location with **GREEN vet wrap.**

The red wrap means, "NOT READY TO GO HOME," **and** the green wrap means, "READY TO GO HOME." We found this to be an easy, efficient way to make sure patients never mistakenly leave with an IV catheter in place.

Parkside Animal Care Center

Green Bay, Wisconsin

Our clients often complained that their dogs would try to lick the incision area after neuters and that the e-collars were a pain to keep on, so we started using testicular blocks for all of our neuters. They've made a significant difference for our clients and their dogs.

Guide Dogs for the Blind Inc.
Boring, Oregon

Have you heard of regulator burnout? Unfortunately, we hadn't either. Our oxygen company delivered new oxygen tanks to our practice. One day, a technician went to turn on the oxygen tank, and, as she was turning the knob on the regulator to open the tank, the regulator exploded, permanently burning and scarring her face. This happens when there is oil on the tank when the regulator is being screwed back on. It's extremely important to keep the area where the tanks are stored very clean and to open the valve on an oxygen regulator very slowly.

Mid-Island Animal Hospital
Hicksville, New York

We place a cork
in each end of our rebreathing tubes.
This way we prevent the escape of
ANESTHETIC GAS
into the room so staff doesn't BREATHE it in,
and particles in the air don't settle in our clean tubes,
ensuring they stay clean.

Multnomah County Animal Services
Troutdale, Oregon

We use COMPLEMENTARY AND ALTERNATIVE MEDICINE to help our patients recover from surgery. Our trained team member sits QUIETLY and centers herself by paying attention to her breath, allowing for longer exhalation than inhalation. She continues this meditative breathing and ENVISIONS A LOVING EXPERIENCE. While holding this loving feeling with a relaxed breath, she places one hand over the sacrum, heart, or kidneys of the sedated patient as he or she AWAKES from anesthesia; the other hand can be used to pet or gently stroke the patient for reassurance. She continues until the patient is through the initial dysphoria, agitation, and fear of the anesthetic experience and can be ambulatory on his or her own. We find it also helps to do this type of procedure in a QUIET SETTING.

Harmony Veterinary Center

Arvada, Colorado

When we would RECONCILE OUR DRUG LOGS, we found that a typical pill counting tray was **too small** and made it too easy to miscount pills, so we CUT A HOLE INTO A LUNCH TRAY to use for pill counts. Now we can **count the pills** with **plenty of room** and deposit them back into the bottle through the hole.

Stone House Animal Hospital
Topeka, Kansas

To keep our controlled drugs **secure**, we installed a MAGNETIC KEY CARD SYSTEM on the room where we keep them. Each card is INDIVIDUALLY ASSIGNED and **coded with level of access.**

Creature Comforts Animal Hospital
Las Vegas, Nevada

To keep our euthanasia solution **separate** from all of the other controlled drugs, we placed the euthanasia solution in a **pencil pouch**. This way there's NEVER any confusion.

VCA Snohomish Animal Hospital
Snohomish, Washington

We are now able to provide **stem cell therapy** for about HALF THE PRICE that we used to. We **harvest** the cells from the patient and CENTRIFUGE them right here; then we send the unused stem cells off-site to be **stored** and **utilized later**.

Veterinary Medical Center of Long Island
West Islip, New York

Chapter 3

Dentistry

We like to send home a **take-home kit** with every dental patient. It's PERSONALIZED with a thank-you card, toothbrushes, mouth rinse, and pet toothpaste, **all in a pencil pouch.**

Wignall Animal Hospital
Dracut, Massachusetts

We started **STAGING OUR DENTALS IN TWO PARTS.** Part one includes scaling, polishing, full mouth radiographs, and probing and charting. A detailed treatment plan is then made for part two regarding extractions. Staging the dentals in two parts allows us to **SCHEDULE EFFECTIVELY AND EFFICIENTLY**, and it allows our **CLIENTS TO SPACE OUT PAYMENTS**. Typically we schedule part two at time of pickup from part one. This has resulted in increased compliance from our clients for dental procedures.

Celtic Creatures Veterinary Clinic Ltd.
Sydney, Nova Scotia, Canada

We organize all our dental prophy supplies in plastic drawers that are labeled based on **DIFFERENT TYPES OF DENTALS**, e.g., small animal dental pack, large animal dental pack. When we are setting up for the dental, we just pull out the appropriate drawer and everything is ready for us: **STERILIZED INSTRUMENTS, PASTE, ANGLE**, etc.

Tara Animal Hospital Inc.
Colleyville, Texas

To HELP all of our staff BETTER UNDERSTAND what is involved in a **dental prophy**, we mixed crushed corn flakes and a sticky substance and put it on a skull's teeth to simulate tartar. After the mixture had hardened, we invited every team member to "CLEAN" the teeth. The staff enjoyed this learning experience.

Hope Springs Veterinary at Great Bridge
Chesapeake, Virginia

To make sure everyone on staff is wearing the **APPROPRIATE PPE (personal protective equipment)** during dental procedures, we have **dental procedure PACKS** that consist of a disposable gown, bonnet or cap, face shield, and eye shield—each individually bagged.

Whenever we have a dental scheduled, **TEAM MEMBERS** just grab a pack and some gloves and **are ready to go.**

Montrose Animal Hospital

Marietta, Georgia

Chapter 4

Radiographs

OUR
radiopaque markers
were constantly being
LOST and MISPLACED,
SO we put them all on a **lanyard**
to keep that from happening.

Markham Animal Clinic Ltd.
Markham, Illinois

We discovered that our new digital X-ray machine will not take a radiograph until we have COMPLETED all the fields, which includes the RIGHT AND LEFT MARKERS. When we called the manufacturer about it, we were told that AN X-RAY IS A LEGAL DOCUMENT, and, as such, the markers must be placed PRIOR to the radiograph being taken. To try and place them after the fact would be ALTERING A LEGAL DOCUMENT. Now, we're glad the machine has this feature.

Palo Verde Animal Hospital

Phoenix, Arizona

We are able to avoid being EXPOSED to **radiation** while taking radiographs by SUFFICIENTLY RESTRAINING all our **PATIENTS.** We are able to use either a CHEMICAL RESTRAINT, the pet's moribund state, or **proper positioning techniques with sandbags and tape**. We find by doing these things, we get a **BETTER-QUALITY IMAGE IN LESS TIME,** and we INCREASE SAFETY AND DECREASE STRESS for both the **patient** and the **staff** member.

Willowdale Animal Hospital

Willowdale, Ontario, Canada

Chapter 5

Euthanasia

When there is a EUTHANASIA APPOINTMENT, instead of hanging signs or trying to tell everyone one by one, we **turn off the lights in the pharmacy area.** When those lights are off, everyone knows not to talk loudly, laugh, or do anything else that might disturb our patients and clients.

Windmill Animal Hospital
Abilene, Texas

When we have a euthanasia appointment, we announce "CODE GREEN" over the PA system, so every staff member is aware and knows to **keep noise down in the hallways and treatment area.**

Markham Animal Clinic Ltd.
Markham, Illinois

At our hospital,
instead of calling our
dedicated euthanasia room a
"comfort room," we call it our

"circle of life room"

because we have delivered
puppies in there, too!

Harlingen Veterinary Clinic

Belle Mead, New Jersey

WE set up our COMFORT ROOM to resemble a **BEDROOM.** It even has a **"bed,"** made of a framed wooden platform with a **plastic-covered MATTRESS** on it. OUR CLIENTS seem to find the room a **soothing and peaceful place** to spend their last moments with **THEIR PETS.**

VCA Village Animal Hospital

Palm Bay, Florida

Chapter 6

Patient Comfort

We came up with a great way to help DE-STRESS CATS during exams and even blood draws. We place the cat in a high-sided litter box with a blanket that has a pheromone product sprayed on it. This has made a BIG DIFFERENCE for the cats, clients, and staff members, especially with blood draws.

Columbia Animal Clinic PC
Brooklyn, Michigan

Our hospital remodeled one of the offices right off the main waiting area into a cat waiting room. We installed soft lighting in the room and decorated it like a living room. By adding a separate waiting room for cats, we not only can be called a "CAT-FRIENDLY PRACTICE," but we've also helped our clients and, most importantly, the cats feel more comfortable. Clients also say their CATS SEEM TO BE CALMER and more relaxed by the time they have their exam.

Bethany Animal Hospital
Sycamore, Illinois

We've set up our exam rooms to have A PEACEFUL AMBIANCE for both dogs and cats. The canine rooms have therapeutic memory foam dog beds and a basket full of toys so they can RELAX OR PLAY. The feline rooms also have a basket of toys, a cat bed by the window, and a hiding place designed to HELP THE CATS FEEL SECURE while still allowing team members to reach them safely. Naturally, we disinfect the beds and toys.

Harmony Veterinary Center
Arvada, Colorado

We have been trying to work on the perception that clients have about it being DIFFICULT to bring their pets to the veterinary hospital. To better combat this PERCEPTION, we've been working on different handling and restraint techniques as well as CHANGING SOME THINGS like lighting, scents, and noise in the hospital.

Willowdale Animal Hospital
Willowdale, Ontario, Canada

We've started using SOUND MACHINES in our exam rooms. We've found that this helps to CALM and SOOTHE the patients as well as the clients. It also helps filter out noise made by passing staff members.

Orchard Road Animal Hospital
Montgomery, Illinois

We decided to use **mini marshmallows** as treats for our dogs with **allergies.** They work **GREAT** as pill pockets and the dogs **LOVE THEM!**

Carmel Veterinary Clinic
Carmel, Indiana

To further protect any animals staying overnight, we installed a device called a **Knox Box** on the outside of our building that allows the local fire department to GAIN ACCESS in the event of an emergency as opposed to having to break the door or windows. The **fire department** has a **key** TO THE BOX, which in turn holds a key to the practice.

Hill Country Animal Hospital
Helotes, Texas

We installed an underwater treadmill recently and HIGHLY RECOMMEND that other practices thinking of doing so have the treadmill FACE the **windows and high-traffic areas**. Otherwise, the dogs spend all their time on the treadmill trying to turn around to see what's behind them.

VCA South Shore Animal Hospital #154
South Weymouth, Massachusetts

Chapter 7

Employee Morale and Training

Some of our employees were concerned with the lack of healthy snack choices available at work. Our medical director found a NUTRITIONIST who was employed by the local supermarket and, for a small fee ($5.00/person), would shop for HEALTHY FOODS and even DELIVER THEM to the practice. To further encourage each other, the team came up with healthy eating tips and hung them and other resources around the break room.

Animal Family Veterinary Care Center
Davenport, Iowa

To encourage some FESTIVE TEAM FUN, we held a pumpkin decorating contest during Halloween. We placed a ballot box at the reception desk along with blank pieces of paper. Each pumpkin had a number in front of it, and we invited clients to VOTE FOR THEIR FAVORITE PUMPKIN. The person who designed the winning pumpkin received a goody basket and a gift card, and we had fun TALKING AND LAUGHING about the designs.

Shady Brook Animal Hospital
Magnolia, Texas

To make SAFETY more **FUN, our safety coordinator designed FUNNY SIGNS** and posted them in key places to remind the team about IMPORTANT SAFETY CONCERNS. They cover topics relating to PROPER HANDLING, ANESTHESIA, RADIOLOGY, and more.

Greenland Veterinary Hospital

Greenland, New Hampshire

Our **hospital manager** has every new employee take the "POLICY MANUAL SCAVENGER HUNT." It's a nice way to say "quiz," but it's fun during your first week of hire. There are roughly **twenty questions** THAT TEST COMPREHENSION of various policies and procedures from our hospital's **employee handbook**, along with SCENARIO QUESTIONS such as, "Mrs. Jones called to request a drop-off euthanasia, as the family dog bit her son last night. How do you schedule this appointment?"

Sunnyvale Veterinary Clinic
Sunnyvale, California

OUR PRACTICE MANAGER created FLASH CARDS, and now they are part of every new hire's orientation packet. The flash cards include medical terminology, common abbreviations, and frequently prescribed medications along with the medications' contraindications, alternate names, and indications. New hires find THESE CARDS TO BE HELPFUL, and we find they onboard more QUICKLY.

Doctors Pet Clinic
Murrieta, California

A 360-degree review benefits employees by helping them understand where they are SUCCESSFUL and where they need to focus additional attention, and services like Survey Monkey allow us to conduct them EFFICIENTLY. The Survey Monkey fee pays for itself in the TIME SAVED by having the information compiled and collated electronically. The software also makes it easy to modify the review forms. We also use this service to do CLIENT SURVEYS.

South Carolina
Veterinary Emergency Care
Columbia, South Carolina

We recently started using a **DOCUMENT management system.** EVERY STAFF MEMBER is required to log on every day to see any **NEW or UPDATED** forms, protocols, and procedures. We have found that this **software has CUT DOWN** on the use of PAPER AND THE SPACE NEEDED to store it all as well as help us **keep track** of which staff members have viewed or signed important documents.

Michigan City Animal Hospital

Michigan City, Indiana

Chapter 8

Client Service and Education

Our clinic installed a stoplight in the treatment area to make us more aware of the noise level. The light tracks the noise level, and when it is getting noisy in the treatment area, the light turns yellow. When it is too loud, the light turns red.

Animal Emergency Hospital of Mansfield
Mansfield, Texas

We've instituted the "10 and 5 rule" for greeting clients as well as fellow staff members. Our rule is to acknowledge the presence of another person within ten feet and verbally greet him or her within five feet. The rule is meant to encourage positive interactions. After discussing the 10 and 5 rule and the importance of positive body language at a staff meeting, we added it to our employee manual. It helps set the tempo for the day, and we have received positive feedback from our clients as well.

Larchmont Animal Clinic
Los Angeles, California

We recognized a need for people to have multiple modes to **schedule appointments**. Our web designer DEVELOPED AN APP that has an appointment request calendar and added more INTERESTING **features** such as breaking news, pet food recalls, and prescription refill requests. It also coordinates with a **click-through button** for scheduling appointments on our website and social media sites. All communications are directed to the client service email. It's not for all of our clients, but the **group of clients** who would MUCH RATHER send a text than pick up the phone **use it frequently**.

Veterinary Associates of Cape Cod Corp.
South Yarmouth, Massachusetts

OUR VETERINARIANS start each day by going through our **appointment schedule** thoroughly. It stems from our desire to respect our clients' time in an effort to provide exceptional client service; EVERY SECOND COUNTS and can be **utilized** TO THE FULLEST when we are prepared.

Willowdale Animal Hospital

Willowdale, Ontario, Canada

● ● ● ● ● ●

We recommend **farm visits** for high-strung working dog breeds that might be developing **behavioral problems** due to boredom. A local farm allows "GUEST HERDERS" to come and work with the sheep and cows. Many clients have stated their dogs seem to love the **exercise**, INTERACTION, **and mental stimulation** that come from HERDING with qualified supervision.

Petaluma Veterinary Hospital

Petaluma, California

We had a **Facebook contest** featuring our patients, and the **winning photos** were printed to display on our walls. The runners-up, along with other photos of our patients, were used to CREATE **a photo mosaic**. We have found that clients love to search for their own pets' pictures in the image.

Mueller Pet Medical Center
Sacramento, California

We have a **whiteboard** in our lobby on which we write every patient's name for the day, WELCOMING THEM TO THE PRACTICE. The clients enjoy seeing their **pets' names** on the board when they come in.

VCA Animal Health Center
Clifton Park, New York

To help with client education, we put out DIGITAL **PICTURE FRAMES in the waiting area** and each **exam room** that display PowerPoint slides on topics such as **SENIOR wellness** and twice-yearly **wellness exams.** We change the images and slides about every three months.

Stack Veterinary Hospital

Syracuse, New York

We collected information on PREVENTIVE HEALTH CARE for adult dogs and cats, printed and framed them, and placed them in all of our EXAM ROOMS and in the lobby for a CREATIVE way to display this valuable information.

Markham Animal Clinic Ltd.
Markham, Illinois

To INCREASE COMPLIANCE with **follow-up appointments** and subsequent preventive health visits, our veterinarians now schedule appointments with clients **before** THEY LEAVE. A veterinarian is in the best position to explain to a client why an appointment is necessary and what will be needed for it and should **book the appointment** with confidence, as if **prescribing** it.

Willowdale Animal Hospital
Willowdale, Ontario, Canada

Chapter 9

Marketing and Public Relations

We set up a **children's veterinary education room** in our practice. The children can DRESS UP like surgeons, VENTILATE a patient, and PERFORM a mock C-section on a dog. **Every MORNING,** one of the receptionists places a TINY **stuffed puppy** into the opening of a stuffed dog; **THEN the kids** PERFORM SURGERY by removing the puppy and even **get to keep it.**

Country Hills Pet Hospital

Eden, Wisconsin

We like to showcase what we have done for the community on a wall in the lobby area, whether it is **raising money for** HOMELESS **pets** or **helping** WILDLIFE. We feel it's a great way to let our clients know that WE ENJOY **being part of the community** and that we are here for **more than just caring** for their best friends.

Wignall Animal Hospital
Dracut, Massachusetts

When we **OPENED FOR BUSINESS**, we decided to run some **fun** promotional events to get the word out about us. In the month of May, we held **"Stinko de Mayo"** instead of Cinco de Mayo and offered **DISCOUNTS ON FECALS** for the whole month. We advertised the promo on our **SOCIAL MEDIA** sites and ended up with 45 fecals that month.

Animal Medical Center of Chandler
Chandler, Arizona

We recently started our own BLOOD BANK for our area and will ship blood products to other hospitals, too. To promote this service, we TEAMED UP WITH THE RED CROSS AND HELD A HUMAN AND PET BLOOD DRIVE at our hospital; while the humans were GIVING BLOOD with the Red Cross, the pets were giving blood with us!

NorthStar VETS

Robbinsville, New Jersey

We used KNOWTHIS.COM when we were developing our marketing plan. We loved having **quick access to recommendations and suggestions** on the ever-changing field of marketing. Marketing spans so many areas and is so fluid, it's ESSENTIAL to have multiple print and digital resources to reference.

South Carolina Veterinary Emergency Care
Columbia, South Carolina

Feline visits were down at our clinic, so we've instituted **"Feline Fridays"** where we offer a discount for feline exams and promote it on our Facebook page and in our office. It's been successful, **bringing in patients** WE HADN'T SEEN IN A WHILE and, in some cases, allowing us to **uncover** and **treat** underlying disease processes.

Animal Medical Clinic of Gulf Gate
Sarasota, Florida

We've added what we call

"CATURDAYS."

The appointments from 8:00 a.m. to 10:30 a.m. on the **first two Saturdays** of the month are for CATS ONLY. That way **no dogs** come into the hospital while the cats are here. It has GONE OVER **VERY WELL** with our clients and their cats, and the appointment slots are almost always FULL.

Bethany Animal Hospital

Sycamore, Illinois

Chapter

10

AAHA Accreditation

As we were preparing for accreditation, one of our DOCTORS made a PowerPoint presentation called **"What's AAHAppening"** to get the whole team involved. It HIGHLIGHTED which of the **recommended PRACTICES** we were already doing and which still needed to be IMPLEMENTED. It ended up being the first in a series of similar presentations.

Advanced Veterinary Care

Farmington, Connecticut

During new-hire orientations, **every NEW employee** is required to watch the *AAHA 101* video and then take a quiz on the information. One such question is, "The Gardner Animal Care Center is held accountable to more than how many standards?" This way EVERY **team member** is educated about AAHA and can speak of the importance of being an AAHA-accredited practice.

Gardner Animal Care Center

Gardner, Massachusetts

As we were getting ready for our AAHA evaluation, we CREATED A **bulletin board** in the staff lounge displaying information about the Standards as a reminder of WHAT WE PRACTICE EVERY DAY.

Hulen Hills Animal Hospital
Fort Worth, Texas

To prepare for our evaluation and get everyone involved, we came up with the idea of playing **AAHA trivia.** We printed out the Standards, cut them up, and put them in a bag. At staff meetings, each team member would have to CHOOSE A **Standard** out of the bag randomly and explain the meaning of it to the whole team. If we were correct, we would receive one "DOGGIE DOLLAR," and after we accumulated ten "doggie dollars," we could trade them in for a ten-dollar gift card to a local business.

Evans Animal Hospital
Evans, Georgia

To PREPARE FOR **AAHA accreditation,** our practice manager assigned different categories in the Standards to **our staff.** In small groups, we had to **PREPARE PRESENTATIONS** on our assigned category to give to the entire staff. SOME GROUPS used PowerPoint presentations while others used storyboards. It was a **GREAT way for everyone** TO WORK TOGETHER and learn about the Standards, even those outside our normal areas of expertise.

Hope Springs Veterinary at Great Bridge

Chesapeake, Virginia

To make learning the **AAHA STANDARDS fun and involve everyone** for our FIRST evaluation, we split into teams and partitioned the **Standards** among the teams. Then we made a CUTE bulletin board divided into tracks with **each track representing a Standard.** Each standard had a marker shaped like a dog that MOVED along the track as the team progressed on the Standard.

Country Doctor Veterinary Hospital

New Tripoli, Pennsylvania